Good Medicine

C. Lloyd Thompson

ISBN-10:1983939307
ISBN-13:9781983939303

DEDICATION

To those of us seeking healing and rejuvenation. I share my research
and experimentation; extracting an essence for others to work with
and find some hope in hopeless conditions.

CONTENTS

ACKNOWLEDGMENTS

To all those who have gone before me.

Those who have taken the time and energy to leave some clues.

Some of them lived solitary lives

Hermits and recluses

Some of them help unseen;
transcended immortals.

We are grateful.

In the course of teaching and sharing my Chi Kung practice with others topics often drift towards nutrition and herbal supplements. Diet can be a polarizing topic for many. It can have the volatility of politics and religion. People are radically committed to their dietary practices or the lack thereof.

I have gone through many changes exploring possible diet and lifestyle changes

I believe the practice of Medicinal and martial Chi Kung has vastly improved my digestion. In the Ayurvedic traditions there are some Tantrics and Aghoris that say, "What you eat is not as important as what you can fully digest.

This is in reference to the three Doshas; Kalpha, Pitta and Vatta. At the end of this book I will include some charts with basic Dosha information. I also correlate the Doshas into a seasonal chart along with the 5-elements for cross-reference.

Since I refer to my system as Tantric Kundalini I also correlate that into the 12 meridians and 8 vessels.

My interest in useful herbs began early on as an outdoors type person; camping, hiking and fishing. I have always been interested in plants with food and medicinal value. I considered it a pastime. I see it as the spirituality of nature; God as expressed in nature.

Astragalus:

anti-bacterial

anti-inflammatory

adaptogen

protects liver

HBP

energy

immunity

detox lungs and spleen

the king of immuno-stimulants

When I was diagnosed with an untreatable form of Leukemia this is one of the first herbs my web search brought me to. I was quite desperate and had zero skillful means as to dosage and consumption.

I bought a large bag of fresh ground root. I cooked it in dosage like I would a regular tea. It almost took my head off. I see why they say it is a naturally occurring plant-based steroid. I felt like I had overdosed on steroids.

Rule number one; brewing raw root is impossible to gauge dosage.

Rule number two; respect all drugs in herb form.

I have been experimenting with dosage in powdered capsule form because the dosage is already measured out.

I have also tried Astragalus in combination with other herbs. My current daily dosage is to break one capsule of 400mg and pour one third to one half of that into the tip of a spoon of raw Reichi mushroom with a spoon of instant coffee in the morning. Sometimes I repeat, depending on what is going on with conditions. I think it has a very rich taste and is a good way to start my day before I do my morning Chi Kung exercises.

Perhaps my early experimenting overdoses were like herbal-chemo therapy. It didn't harm me other than discomfort.

Ashwaganda:

Indian Ginseng

deep sleep induce

anti-carcinogen

lower cholesterol

memory and brain function

sexual/physical strength

sidhis

clairvoyance

This was the second major healing herb I picked up. I liked the fact that it was listed as an aphrodisiac herb. I had zero sexual function at that time. I could force and erection with Viagra. Underneath was pure impotence along with erectile dysfunction.

I did the same thing with this herb. I bought a bag of raw root and brewed it up strong like a decoction. I probably had a 100xs overdose compared to what I later used in ongoing therapy.

I went wheelin my bike all over the city like I was in my 20s. "Wow. I like this feeling." The aging body paid a price for jet fuel exertion. Nothing was broken, torn or damaged. But....I was soooo stiff and sore later.

No significant increase in sexual performance other than wishful thinking about all the hot women I saw. They didn't seem to notice the lonely old man eyeing them.

What I found that did work was a drastic decrease in social anxiety. I was able to use it before social involvements and stayed somewhat clear.

Fo Ti:

In Chinese Medicine this is one of the herbs that has a mythology all of its own. Stories tell of this being a magic secret from the masters and the temples. It is one of the legendary herbs of longevity.

Chinese Medicine has stories of Taoist hermits who have lived hundreds of years. They speak of immortality being the main goal.

Who doesn't want immortality? Especially if you are staring down the barrel of a terminal diagnosis with no known treatment? So, I began doing some research. Then I did what I usually do. I went to Amazon.com and typed it in to compare products and prices. And, as I usually do, I ordered samples and began my experimentation phase.

Being my own Lab-rat-guinea pig, I learn to watch for signs of adverse reactions with small doses; high blood pressure, anxiety levels and other mental and bodily function for adverse or allergic reactions.

I did as much of it as I could for as long as I could; given that it causes many strange sensations and feelings that weren't painful but not pleasant either.

What good did it do? It seems impossible to do a scientific analysis because there are so many variables involved; and......many of the claims are esoteric and mystical. It's difficult to isolate one element for empirical data analysis.

But.....I can say that when I began using Fo Ti my hair and beard were completely white and grey. I have photos to prove it. It is a sign of aging; especially into my 60s; just a fact of life, if you don't want to use coloring agents, that's it till you die.

Every time I looked it the mirror I could not find one single hair on my face or head that had any color in it. Then I began to notice some black hairs growing in. It's the sort of thing where you rub your eyes and check to see if it's the light.

Is this some kind of a fluke? Or is it some sort of miracle of reversing the aging process? It's been over five years since I first began the Fo Ti experiment.

My beard has many colors in it. My hair is light brown, blondish
with some silver highlights. I grow my beard think and curly and my
hair long just to display the miracle.

Epimedium:

Also known as Horny Goat Weed. Most people in the west think of Epimedium as the Friday night date pill or powder.

In traditional Chinese Medicine it has been prescribed for hundreds of years for ailments related to aging.

I noticed in my research that many of the herbs that held possibility to help me heal my cancer also had a profile as aphrodisiac. That's where I began to ponder my data and consider what it might mean. That's when my research into medicinal Chi Kung led me to the concept of Jing-Chi.

In Chinese medicine and Medicinal Chi Kung the lower tan tien (about 2 or 3 fingers below the navel) is associated with the water element. It is a type of energy reservoir for this water element. This is called Jing-Chi; the regenerative energy of life, also called sexual energy.

In Medicinal Chi Kung men are cautioned to learn semen retention. Ejaculation is a release of semen, which is also Jing-Chi. Men are given skills to have intercourse and experience wonderful orgasms without ejaculation thus conserving the regenerative energy of life and circulating it through the vessels and meridians for health and longevity.

Women are the winners in Medicinal Chi Kung. They can have multiple orgasms including female ejaculation without depleting themselves the way men do. Men are better able to give multiple orgasms and frequent intercourse through the practice of semen retention.

Aphrodisiac herbs and formulas can be a positive factor for increasing sexual energy; thus the possibility of increasing Jing-Chi. The goal is to increase Jing-Chi in the lower reservoir until it begins to overflow into the eight major energy vessels. It's sort of like a reservoir fills up and spills over into irrigation channels. When the eight energy vessels are full to overflowing they spill over into the twelve meridians, which nourish the vital organs.

Epimedium and many aphrodisiac herbs and formulas because the focus of my research and experimentation. I did have some sparks of success. My energy levels improved. My depression lessened. My Eros, libido improved so that I had energy and interest in reaching out and interacting with others.

Dan Shen:

But....some cancers are more stubborn than others. I remember laying on my bed large portions of the day....no energy. I knew it was my deathbed. The lymph glands on my neck were swollen. They felt hot and tender to the touch.

Dan Shen is also known as Red Sage. It is one of the many herbs currently being studied by western medicine. It shows some promise.

I didn't have much to loose if I took it in the wrong dose. The root chips are rock hard. I put them in a clear glass so I could monitor the color as it brewed. I set it on the kitchen counter to brew over night.

I remember looking in the morning to see a long black line from the glass to an electrical outlet. It's the kind of thing where you rub your eyes, "What the heck?"

I got up closer and saw that it was a line of black ants pouring out of the light socket and going to drink from the Dan Shen glass.

I have read stories that ancient shaman used to follow bears and other animals to see what herbs they dug up and what they did with it. Many healing herbs were discovered by ancient tribes in this manner.

I know that the ants knew there was something tremendously important to imbibe. And that they could smell it from a long ways off because I had zero ants before my experiment.

I watched the ants with fascination as the brew darkened and their colony got the medicine they needed. The herb has many possibilities. One of them is for nourishing and healing the brain from deterioration and injury such as strokes. I know my brain needed all the help it could get; bad nutrition, drug overdoses and general neglect.

The dosage proved tricky for me. It had a harsh kickback in terms of mood and anxiety, feelings and thoughts from the biochemistry. I began dipping my fingers in the brew and rubbing it directly on my swollen lymph nodes. I could feel some sort of twitching response in the swollen areas. So I began to rub it all over my neck. I rubbed in my armpits and around my eyes also.

I learned later in Medicinal Chi Kung that the brain and spinal column are considered part of the lymph system. I was absorbing Dan Shen directly into my lymph nodes and my brain.

Desperate and dying, I felt like my cancer was at a point where it was ready to explode, catch fire and eat me alive.

I awoke the next morning with the heaviest eye crusts of my life. So much junk was crusted on my eyelids that I could barely make my way to the bathroom to begin rinsing and prying loose the crusts.

It would have been interesting to have taken some of the eye crusts to a lab for analysis. They say not to lick your tears because the tear duct release toxins. I must have been full of toxins.

It was uncomfortable and somewhat embarrassing to be in public

and have my eyes crusting over. Better than exploding with tumors.

Medicinal Mushrooms:

Some cancers are such monsters they have never been conquered, treated or cured. Now matter how soundly you throw them to the matt. They get back up and begin eating at you again.

That was the case with this Leukemia. I knew I had done some massive cleansing. But the cancer creating the mutated cells was still alive and active; generating more mutated cells to be cleansed.

Somewhere deep inside I must have had a desire to live. I didn't feel like sinking quietly into my deathbed. Somewhere inside I heard the whisper, "Your life is just beginning." My decades of learning, experimentation and evolving was about to blossom shine.

My research led me to Medicinal mushrooms. This is an area that has become available to the general public as an indirect result of the experimentation of the 60s with Magic mushrooms; and perhaps the

18

latter day saint.....prophet of Medicinal mushrooms, Paul Staymets.

Western medicine has also been taking a look at Medicinal mushroom. There are over twenty mushrooms with a medicinal potential. Many personal testimonies about miraculous healing from hopeless conditions.

I began my experimentation with a combination of 18 mushrooms. It was suggested to me at the local herb store that I go ahead and take double the recommended dosage, "Just get it over with.", was her comment. There were apparently no contraindication warnings about doubling the dosage. "Look at it as a kind of herbal chemo.", she said.

It was summer time. I was due for my annual vision cleansing camp in the mountains. I went to a semi-private spot in the Siskiyou Mountains. It was next to a clear mountain creek with tall timber all around. Nothing to do but talk to my soul, walk in the woods and take my mushroom therapy. I was doing a partial fast; mostly teas and clean out fruits.

I sat for long periods at a vortex spot I made into a Medicine Wheel. My feet were bare so I could feel the rich mountain soil underneath the moss. It was when I began energy circulation for real.

I visualized my spiral energy roots going deep into the soil. Perhaps the medicine of the Medicinal mushrooms helped me to actually feel the energy rising into my channels and meridians with fresh Earth Chi.

It may have been the first time in my life that I felt connected to the earth. I remembered feeling this when I was a child playing outside.

Breathing in Earth Chi is satisfying to the body, mind and soul. I was experiencing a Medicinal mushroom spiritual awakening. I went to stand barefoot on a large boulder that had been warmed by the sun. I could feel myself absorbing various types of Earth Chi. I knew it was not foreign to me.

I went and sat with my bare feet in the cold mountain creek. It was like having my bare feet in the mountain soil. I could feel a different type of Chi being drawn up into my channels.

I finished the bottle at double dose as recommended by the herbalist lady. I continued to explore with different brands and different mushroom combinations, mostly in regular dosage unless I was having a flare-up.

I went for my routine annual check up which included blood work labs. I explained to the nurse practitioner that I had cancer and the white blood cell count would be high.

When I went in for the results he looked at me quizzically as if to say, "He has no idea what he's talking about." The white blood cell count was normal. I knew from experience that most of western medicine dismisses people like me; outsiders.....non-licensed. So I let him think I had imagined the whole thing. I took my miracle with me.

They did DNA sequencing of my bone marrow when the final diagnosis was done. The cancer doctor told me that nobody that he knew of had ever had success with this type of cancer. It's a slow moving train and you are tied to the tracks.

It is a major miracle. I also know that it is not completely cured. There is still some activity in the marrow that shows up as mild swelling of the glands; but it doesn't create elevated white blood cell count.

It is in relative remission. I still continue most of my successful therapies on a regular basis. They not only help to keep the killer in containment, they are wonderful for overall health and longevity with energy and functionality.

A life without Jing Chi is and open door to predatory diseases, atrophy and degeneration.

Ayurveda:

My studies take me outside the scope of traditional Chinese medicine and Chi Kung as most people teach it. It's roots go back 3,000 to 5,000 years in China. There are also parallel practices from India that also date back about the same.

There was an Indian monk/prince who traveled to the Shaolin temples of China about 525 AD. He was called Bodhisattva or Da Mo, depending on your reference. The legends and myths of who he was and what he did are not important to me.

What's important to me is that he had prior training before he traveled to China. He is credited with creating Zen Buddhism in China and Japan. He also has some credit in Chi Kung and Kung Fu.

Ayurveda comes from the fourth Veda. Some of the traditional caste system leaders don't accept it as a valid Veda because it differs from the other three.

Ayurveda stems from the three Gunas; Tamas, Rajas, and Sattvas. In the westernized versions of Yoga these Gunas are said to relate solely to types of foods and the consciousness and energies they produce when you eat them. This is true. But in the larger scheme of things they have a larger meaning. The three Gunas refer to the three states of evolution.

Actually, everything has a place and time. If you are experiencing an accelerated evolution experience such as Kundalini rising Tamasic food might save your life by slowing things down enough for you to survive.

There is another trinity in Ayurvedic medicine. These are called the Doshas. They are related to types of body constitutions. They also relate to the seasons of the year. So, this is where I am able to line up and correlate the three Doshas with the five elements of Chi Kung on the seasonal change wheel.

The Doshas have some basic correlation to early beginnings of western medicine and Hippocrates, He called them blood humors. Foods and medicines react very differently depending on the person's Dosha constitution. One person's nutrition and or medicine is quite literally another person's poison.

It is said that what you can digest is more important than what you eat. Partially digested foods and energies get trapped in the system. This is called Ama. It is a main source of sicknesses.

One thing that I experience from intense practice of Chi Kung is a greatly improved digestive process. The qualities and characteristics of your bowel movements are one way to tell how thoroughly your food has been digested.

In closing, I include a chart of the Doshas so you can get a feel.

Doshas

Vatta:

Season: late fall

Humor: Wind

movement and circulation

calming and warming to balance

Spices:

licorice

ginger

cardamon

cinnamon

sarsaparilla

anise

fennel

clove

stevia

Herbal teas:

rosebuds, chamomile, spearmint, lemon grass, tulsi and orange

Kalpha:

Season; Late fall, early winter

Humor; Lubrication

Phlegm, mucous

stimulating to balance

Spices:

ginger

clove

black pepper

cardamon

tumeric

safron

Pitta:

Season: Late spring, early summer

Humor: Bile

digestion

Cooling to balance

Spices:

cardamom

licorice

ginger

cinnamon

cabbage

rose petals

Herbal teas:

hibiscus, chamomile, peppermint, red rose petals

Gunas:

Evolutionary states:

Tamas; inert, un-manifest matter, consciousness is everything,

Shiva

Rajas; activity, Goddess, Shakti,

Kali

Sattva; self-realization, Shiva/Shakti union,

Shiva as self

Guna foods:

Tamas; heavy, hard to digest

Rajas; bitter, sour, salty, hot, increase activity

Sattva; fresh, light, sweet, bliss

ABOUT THE AUTHOR

If you would like to leave comments for the author

or for other readers

you may do so at:

lordshivakalima.tumblr.com